What is CBD - The Truth about Cannabidiol - Medication

By:

Ray Tokes

I0439614

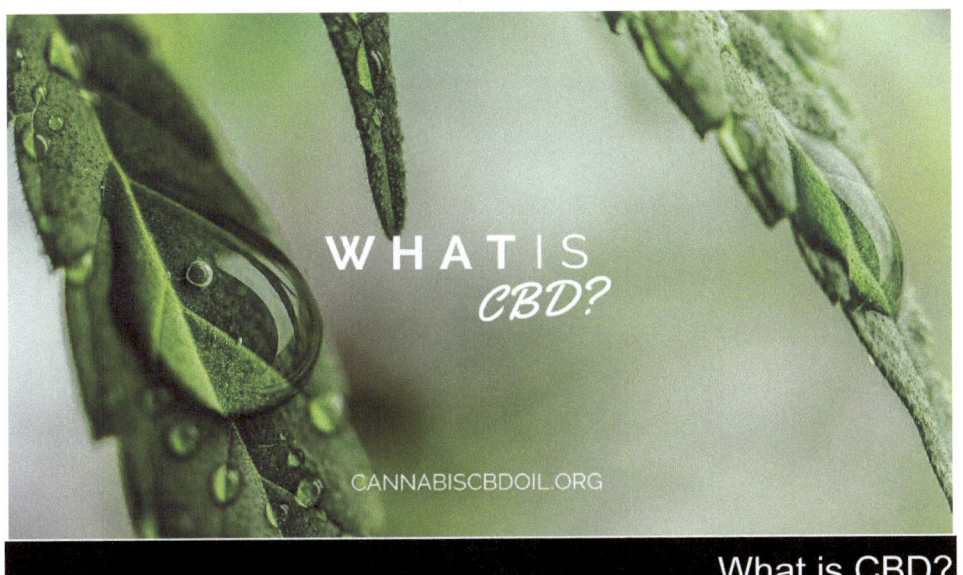

There is still a considerable amount of mystery surrounding CBD. What is it? Where does it come from? Is it legal? Why do people like it so much? These are all important questions. I will provide answers to all of them throughout this book. The information provided will be based on hard fact, rather than conjecture. It will offer a balanced and practical view of CBD, so that readers are able to make an informed choice about whether or not it is right for them.

So, first things first, what is CBD? Most people are aware that it has something to do with the cannabis plant. This is what causes the most confusion and unease, but getting an unbiased perspective is the key to dispelling anxiety. CBD, cannabidiol, is derived from the whole cannabis plants, but is not the same as THC. THC is the component that produces the 'high'.

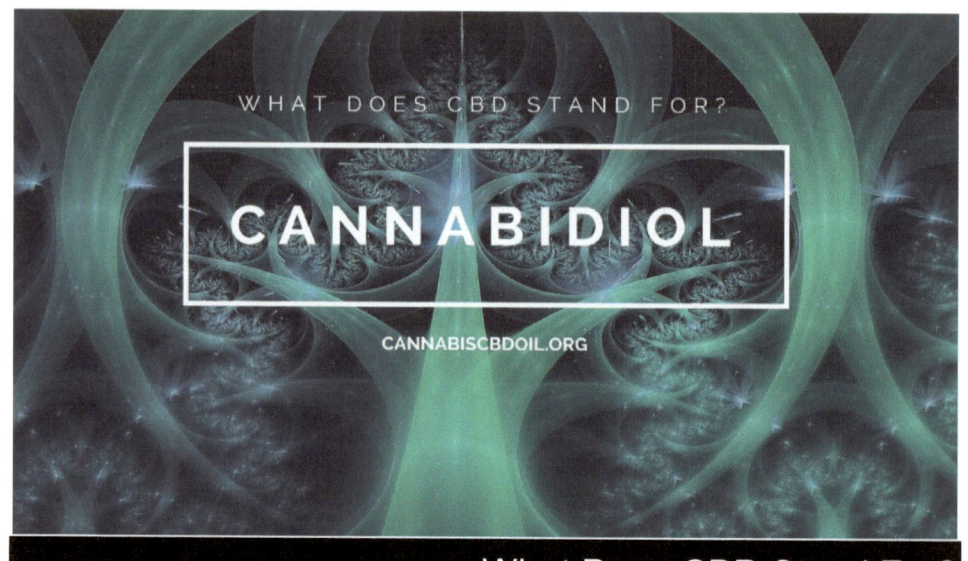

The term CBD is simply an abbreviation for cannabidiol. This is a natural substance that is taken from cannabis (hemp) plants. It has a wide range of different uses and can be employed as everything from a dietary supplement to an anti-anxiety treatment, a pain reliever, and much more. While the benefits of CBD are huge, its association with the cannabis plant means that these capacities are yet to be fully explored.

With every passing year, however, the attitude towards CBD softens. As the science behind its remarkable powers grows, so too does the level of interest in it. In recent years, it has become an increasingly acceptable means of relief for anxiety and inflammation. It is important to understand that CBD is not the same as THC. While THC is mostly illegal, CBD is fully legal in almost every part of the world.

A person cannot get 'high' from ingesting CBD. If they buy a cannabidiol product, it will not alter their state of mind in the same way as smoking cannabis. While studies have shown that it can ease tension and worry, it does not affect the body or the mind in the same way. People interested in trying CBD should remember this distinction when they next come to consider investing in a CBD product.

Where does
CBD
COME FROM?

Where Does CBD Come From?

CBD is extracted and separated from specific strains of cannabis (known as hemp plants). Chemically, it is one of 85 chemical compounds referred to as 'cannabinoids.' These are all found in cannabis plants. However, CBD is the second most common compound, with THC being the most common. In a typical plant, CBD makes up for around 40% of the cannabinoid extracts contained inside.

THC and CBD is not the same thing, so they cannot be used in the same way. In fact, CBD develops in a completely different manner to THC. The two compounds are completely separated and isolated within the plant. CBD high hemp contains only the tiniest traces of THC. This amount is so small that it cannot be regulated, nor is there any point trying to do so. A person cannot get high from consuming CBD oil products either (they do not contain THC).

CBD is extracted in the form of oil. It is usually combined with hemp oil extracts and can be bought in a variety of concentrations. It can be bought and ingested it legally, but it is important to be an informed consumer. Shoppers should know what they want before they buy. They need to make sure that they always buy from reputable sellers.

Finally, they need to be aware that cannabidiol is still a very new product. Due to a reluctance on the part of scientists and researchers to fully investigate its benefits (though this is slowly changing), there are still only a handful of studies on its use. Therefore, consumers of CBD should do their own research before deciding to make these products a regular part of their lives.

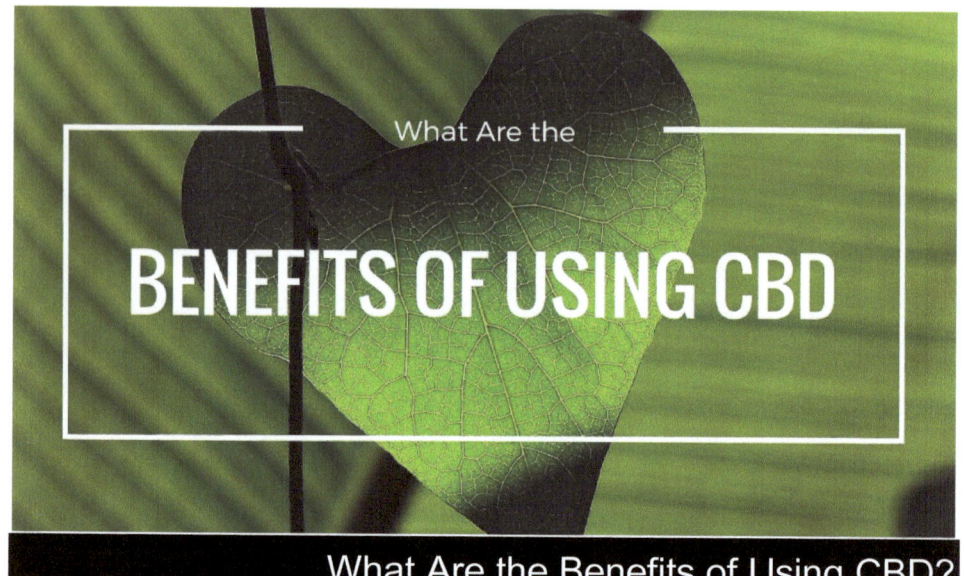

What Are the Benefits of Using CBD?

Over the last decade, there has been compelling evidence to suggest that CBD can alleviate a wide variety of symptoms. Its benefits have been linked with everything from epilepsy to multiple sclerosis, muscle spasms, anxiety disorders, bipolar disorder, schizophrenia, chronic nausea, convulsions, inflammation, and cancer.

There is a lot of evidence and it is extremely convincing. However, almost all of it still needs to be backed up by thorough scientific research. As aforementioned, the attitude of the medical community needs to change before this can happen. The good news is that positive developments are being made, so CBD is likely to appear in a lot more scientific studies over the next five to ten years.

REDUCE

It is widely agreed, by most medical experts, that CBD has the potential to reduce anxiety symptoms. It also slows down the development of aggressive viral strains like the deadly MRSA bug. On the grounds of its chemical makeup alone, it is clear to see that CBD is a very powerful antioxidant. This is a feature that could prove useful for the diet and health industries.

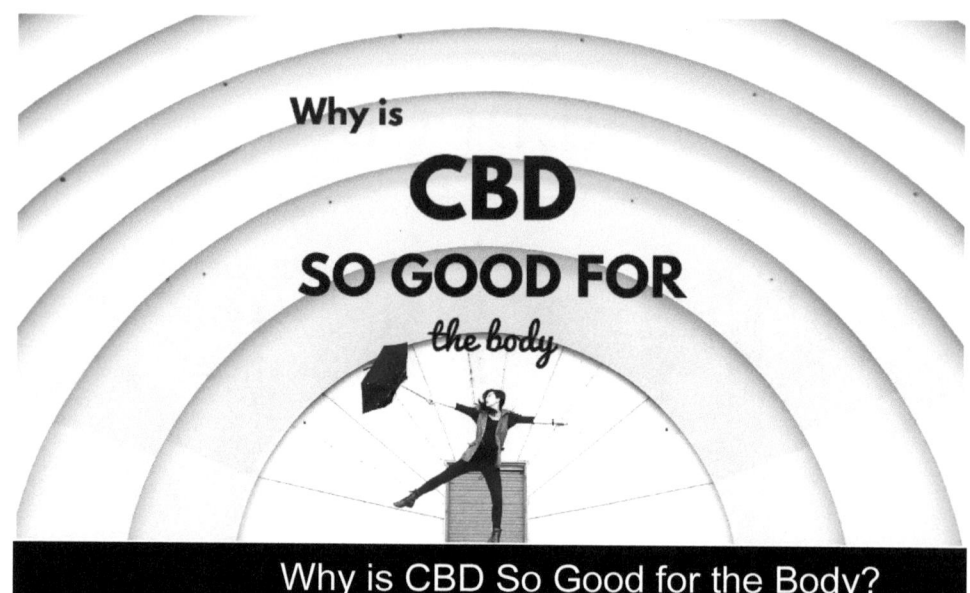

Why is CBD So Good for the Body?

CBD communicates with the cells in the human body, by activating their cannabinoid receptors. In very simple terms, these receptors are responsible for carrying signals. They generate a variety of different physiological consequences. There are some cannabinoid compounds that are not so great for the body. In large enough doses, they can cause depression and a disconnection from reality.

Fortunately, these compounds are very different to CBD. As of yet, there is no scientific evidence to suggest that CBD has any kind of detrimental impact on the body or mind. This is why CBD can be legally sold and distributed. If a person is still nervous or anxious about trying it, they should remember this stone cold fact. It really wouldn't be legal if the regulators could find any reason to prevent or restrict its use.

To return to the cannabinoid receptors, these special signaling sites make up much of the endocannabinoid system. This area of the body controls and regulates things like appetite, pain tolerance, mood, memory, and more. It should be starting to make a little more sense now. CBD is such a powerful substance, because it affects so many different bodily functions.

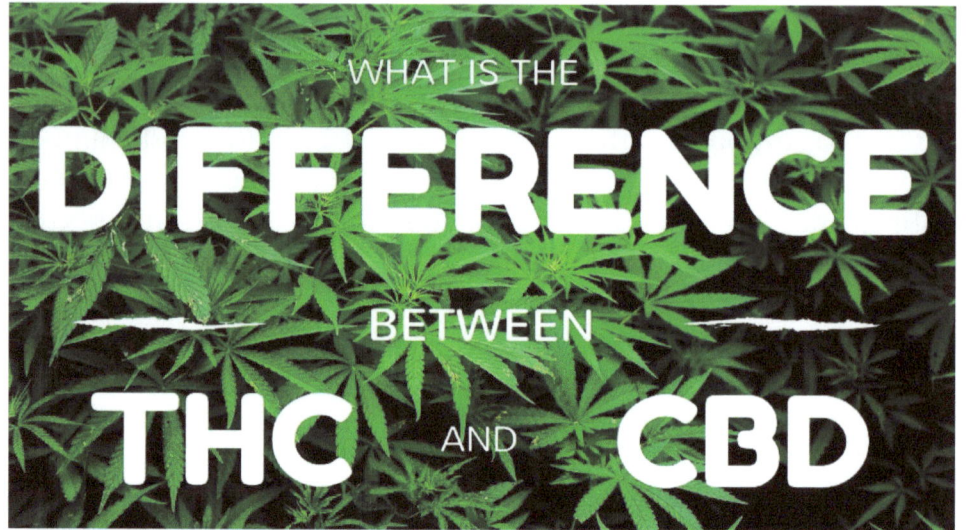

What is the Difference between CBD and THC?

The term CBD as stated, stands for cannabidiol; the term THC stands for tetrahydrocannabinol. These two compounds are the two most commonly found within hemp cannabis plants. They both interact with the cells in the human bodies, but they do so in markedly different ways. While THC is known to get those who ingest it 'high,' CBD does not have this effect on the body.

Though THC and CBD are derived from the same plant and share many molecular similarities, they are distinct. They should not be confused, because this inability to distinguish between the two has already led to CBD products being unfairly restricted. It is possible, however, to legally buy and distribute CBD products in most parts of the world.

A person **cannot legally** buy products that contain THC in most countries. There are exceptions to the rule (with the number increasing every year), but do be aware that it is a strictly controlled and regulated substance. A person should not attempt to buy or distribute products containing THC unless they are sure that their country allows it. In most places, this will not be the case.

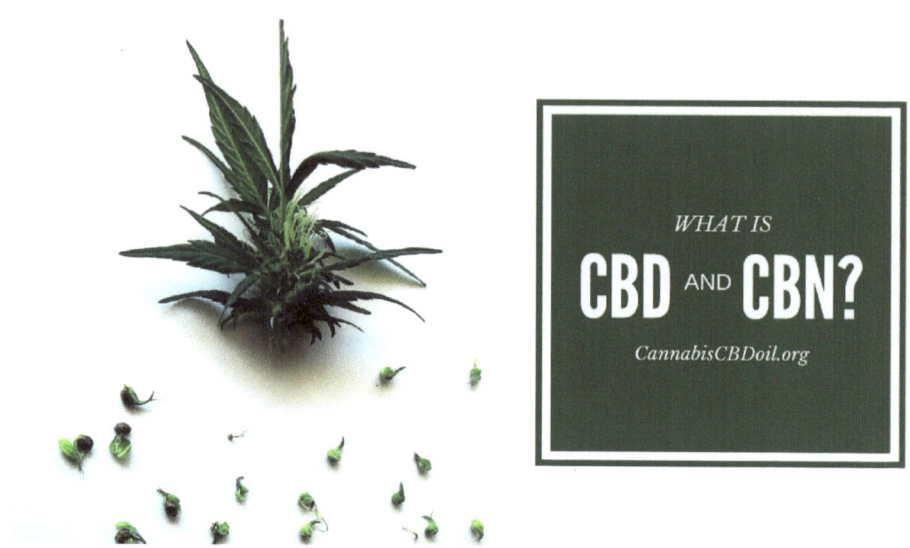

What is the Difference between CBD and CBN?

It is time to introduce another substance. Once again, it is probably clear now why attitudes are so confused about cannabidiol. It can be a confusing topic. With the right advice and information, however, being informed does not have to be a chore. The distinction between CBD and THC should be obvious at this point. Yet, what is the difference between CBD and CBN? Is there a difference?

CBD and CBN **is not the same thing**. CBN is produced when THC matures, ages, and starts to break down. This process is called oxidization. It tends to change the type of high that cannabis smokers feel, so most attempt to avoid or delay it. This can be done by storing cannabis products in a cool, airtight, and dark environment.

Yet, there is evidence to suggest that even CBN has benefits for the body. Do be aware that **it is illegal**, because it contains THC. Nevertheless, it is used by many smokers as a sleep aid and a way to relieve the symptoms of chronic insomnia. CBN is responsible for the sedative like effect of smoking cannabis, so this makes perfect sense.

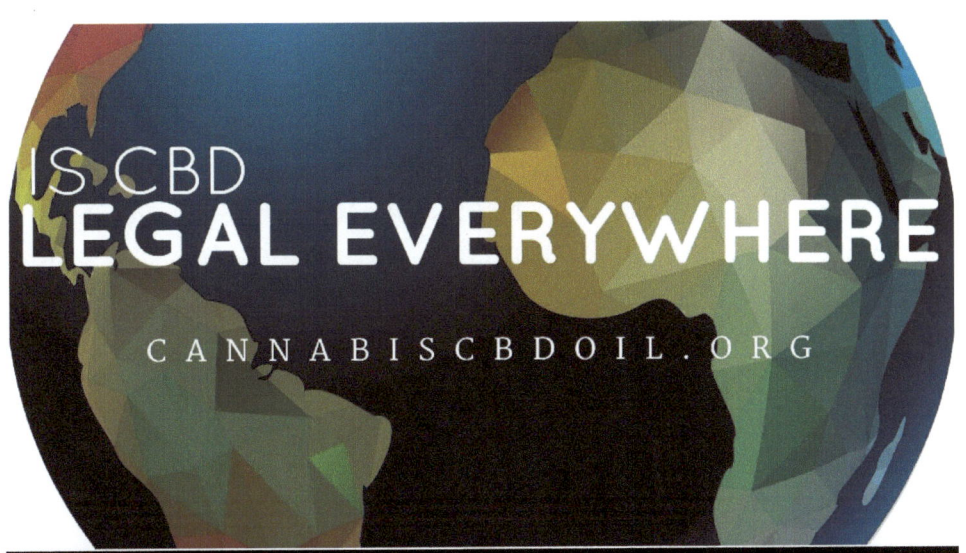

Is CBD Legal Everywhere?

Currently, CBD products are **legal to buy** and distribute in almost every country on the planet. The only prominent exception to this is Canada. In Canada, CBD is a controlled substance. There is no evidence to suggest that it has harmful side effects of any kind. There is also no evidence to suggest that stronger concentrations can be harmful.

Right now, the medical consensus is that CBD can be safely ingested in any amount or concentration. It can be legally sold and used as a dietary supplement. It is usually sold in its natural form, as an oil. To extract this oil, the fatty acids from the stalks of a cannabis plant must be harvested. Inside these fatty acids, there are fat soluble compounds. As cannabinoids are also fat soluble, they leave the plant with the oil.

The problem, for the market, is that the term 'cannabidiol' cannot be easily separated from cannabis. If one hears it, one immediately thinks of cannabis plants, THC, and the illegality of both of these substances. They become one and the same. Yet, in reality, things could not be more different. CBD is distinct from THC, because of its chemical composition.

Even the slightest change to this composition would stop it from being CBD. It cannot be both THC and CBD at the same time. While the former will get you high, the latter is not designed to do this. A person can ingest it safely, without the risk of losing their senses or sense of self. Plus, it has a huge range of medical applications. What is not to love about CBD?

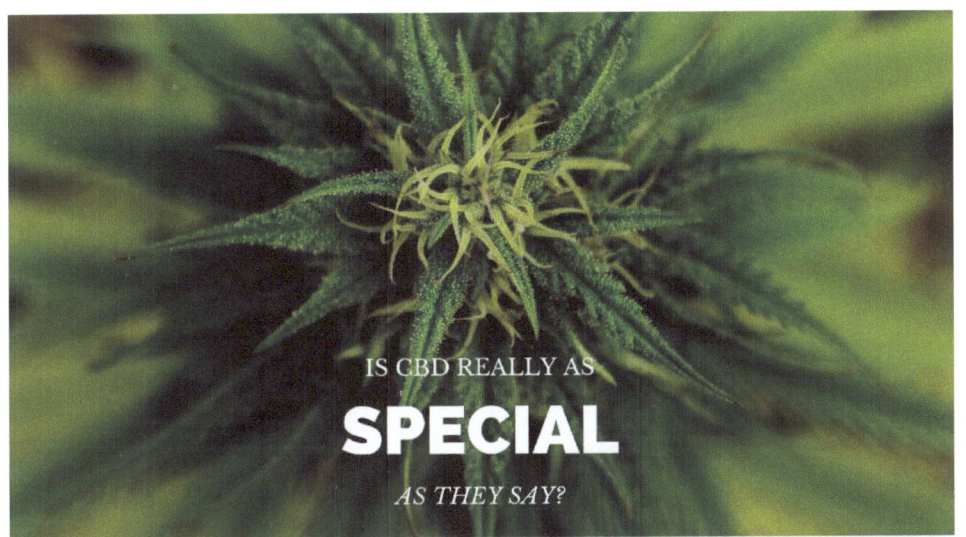

IS CBD REALLY AS

SPECIAL

AS THEY SAY?

Is CBD Really as Special as They Say?

There is only one sure fire way to find out. Trying CBD products, for the first time, can be a really rewarding and satisfying experience. This is especially true for people with medical conditions and chronic anxiety or pain disorders. If traditional medications are not working, CBD oils can offer a natural, body friendly alternative.

Shopping for CBD oils and CBD products needs to be done carefully. There is not a lot of regulation associated with these products, so it is important to research vendors and suppliers before making purchases. It is always worth consulting a doctor for advice if CBD oils are to be used in conjunction with other medications.

Its use is legal, so do not be afraid to discuss it with a specialist. They might be able to give some more in depth information on the best products and vendors. They will also be able to offer advice on whether or not CBD products are likely to have a positive impact on specific symptoms. Though CBD has been linked to the relief of all kinds of disorders and conditions, there are plenty more that it probably has no effect on.

Check online reviews, read testimonials, and only buy from reputable sellers. The CBD oil that is purchased should contain no quantifiable amounts of THC. One of the most popular ways to ingest it is as an e-liquid. It could be worth investing in an e-cigarette device, because e-liquid offers a convenient, quick, and fuss free form of consumption.

For those who intend to use CBD as a dietary supplement, the same rules apply. Shop carefully and be an informed consumer. Treat CBD products in the same way as any dietary aid or supplement. Do not over ingest, combine with a balanced diet and healthy lifestyle, and avoid using as a substitute for good diet and exercise.

Despite a lack of medical research on the benefits of CBD, most scientists and medical experts are very clear on the fact that cannabidiol (CBD) can be extremely friendly to the human body. There is evidence to suggest that it alleviates the symptoms of things like anxiety disorders, convulsions, chronic nausea, arthritis, and even cancer.

If all of these links can be thoroughly tested and backed up by medical studies, CBD promises to revolutionize the medical industry. First though, the stigma surrounding its use needs to go. The term 'cannabidiol' is so close to the term 'cannabis' that, for many decades, scientists have shied away from investigating its use.

For a long time, it was simple assumed that they were the same thing. It was thought that if a person ingests CBD, they might as well be smoking cannabis. Nowadays, this is known to be patently untrue. The chemical cannabidiol compound responsible for getting a person 'high' is THC and CBD could not be more different.

For one thing, CBD cannot get a person high. It does not have this effect on the mind or body. It can calm, soothe, and relax a person, but it does not impair their senses or ability to respond to stimuli. THC and CBD may come from the same plant, but they are distinct. This is why CBD is legal to buy and distribute in almost every country (excepting Canada).

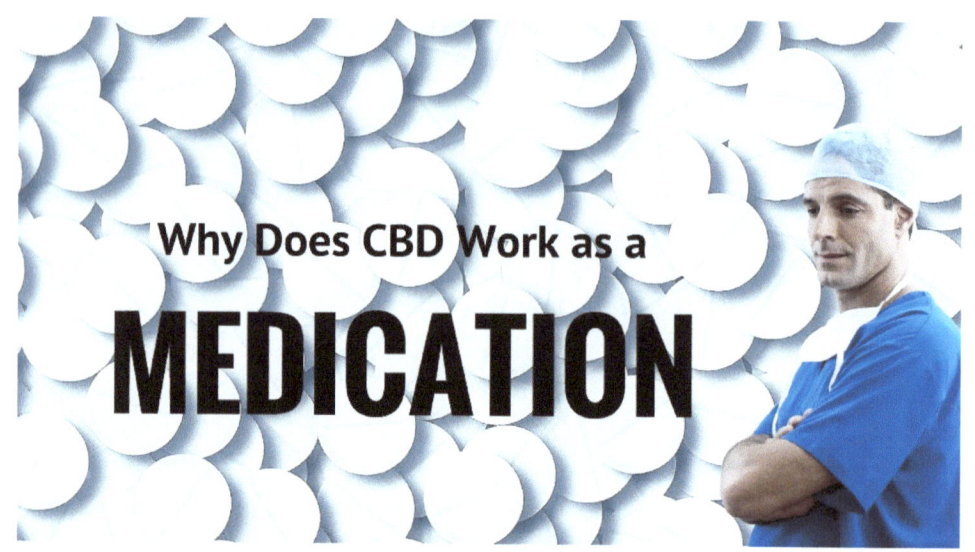

Why Does CBD Work as a MEDICATION

Why Does CBD Work as a Medication?

There are 85 different cannabinoids that scientists have identified. This number includes THC and CBD. These compounds are all different and distinct, though they may interact with one another in certain circumstances and combinations. For example, CBD actually inhibits the psychotropic effects of THC if the two are ingested at the same time.

CBD interacts with the cells in the human body, by 'switching on' their cannabinoid receptors. These receptors carry all kinds of different signals around the body. They are responsible for a huge variety of different functions. By influencing these functions at their place of origin, CBD manages to alter a surprising number of them.

The receptors regulate and control things like appetite suppression, pain tolerance, mood, and memory. Therefore, CBD can potentially influence all of these things. The good news is that there is no evidence to suggest that CBD compounds are harmful in any way. Apart from the fact that they can make people a little sleepy, they seem to only have a positive impact.

This remains the same no matter what concentration they are taken in or how often. However, it is important to remember that medical science is, in many ways, a little backward on this issue. Despite growing evidence to support the medical use of CBD treatments, scientists are still a little squeamish about working with cannabidiol. This taboo is what needs to change if the medical industry is ever to fully explore the benefits of CBD.

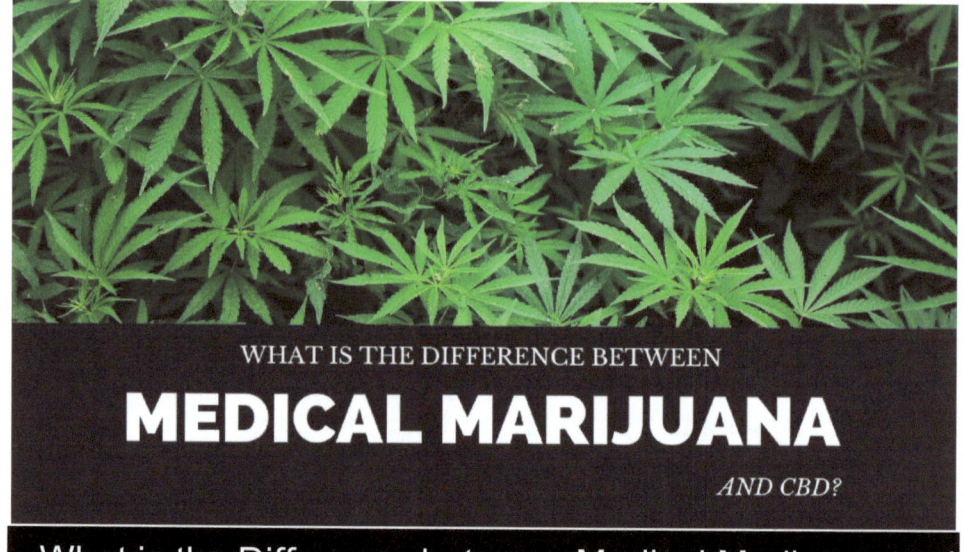

What is the Difference between Medical Marijuana and CBD?

The distinction between medical marijuana and CBD products is the same as the one between CBD and THC. If a person lives in an area or country where it is legal (with a medical licence) to buy or smoke marijuana, they also have the right to ingest medically regulated THC. There is no CBD equivalent, because CBD is legal in most countries.

It can be bought in stores or online from reputable vendors. Even if you do live in a region where medical marijuana is the norm, it is not always the best choice. There are lots of reasons why CBD is superior to THC, especially when it comes to the treatment of medical conditions. For one thing, CBD does not lead to the same kind of paranoia or edginess that THC does.

There is no sensation of being out of control or losing the ability to think clearly. These aspects alone make it the superior choice for most people. Yes, it may make a person feel sleepy, but there are CBD strains that are cultivated specifically to lessen this effect. Plus, sleepiness can be a real advantage for anybody suffering with chronic insomnia or another sleep disorder.

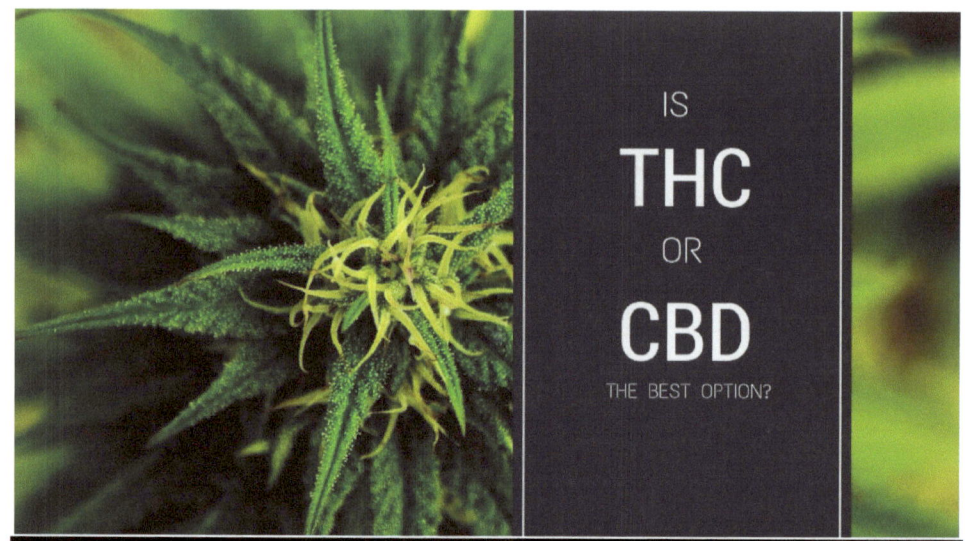

Is THC or CBD the Best Option?

This is a debate that crops up again and again among cannabis and CBD users. The most accurate answer is that CBD is a superior choice for many reasons, but it is also very different to THC. The two are so distinct that it is of less value than most people think to compare them in this way. However, CBD is legal and widely available, so it definitely has the jump on THC.

If a person is not a recreational cannabis smoker (legal or otherwise), CBD is likely to be a wonderful addiction to their daily routine. The only kind of people that often do not find it helpful are heavy cannabis users, because it does not produce a 'high.' Nevertheless, CBD is very safe, can be consumed in strong concentrations, and offers a huge range of medical benefits.

People interested in trying CBD oils or other products for the first time should do their own research on the best places to shop and the best ways to consume it. There is a distinct lack of medical research on the uses of CBD, though the advantages are widely acknowledged, so it is essential to shop smart and be an informed consumer. Work with reputable vendors, know the product, and follow all instructions carefully.

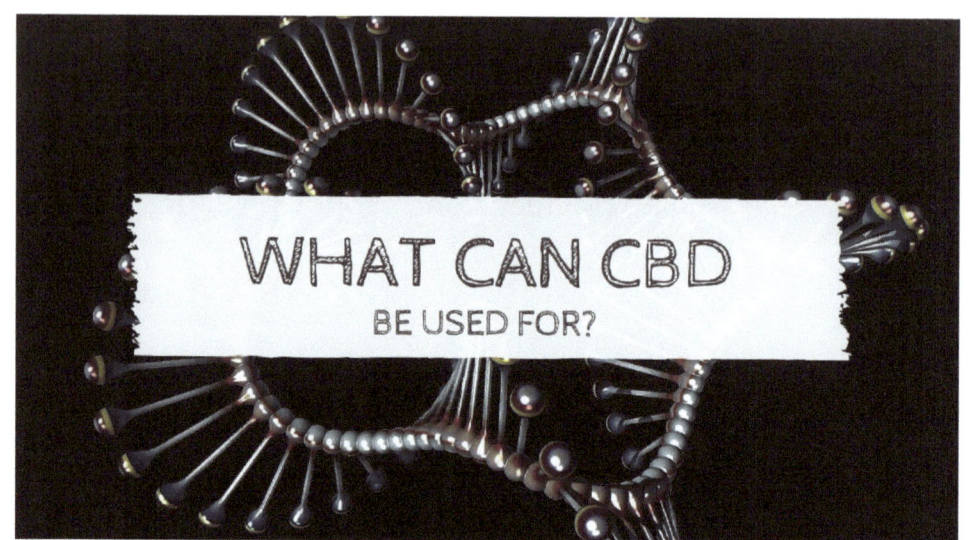

It is time to take a closer look at some of the main uses for CBD oil products. Some are surprisingly and some less so, but all are rather remarkable. The fact that CBD affects the body in such a complex way there are numerous ways that CBD helps the body in a way - regenerate.

Cigarette Addiction

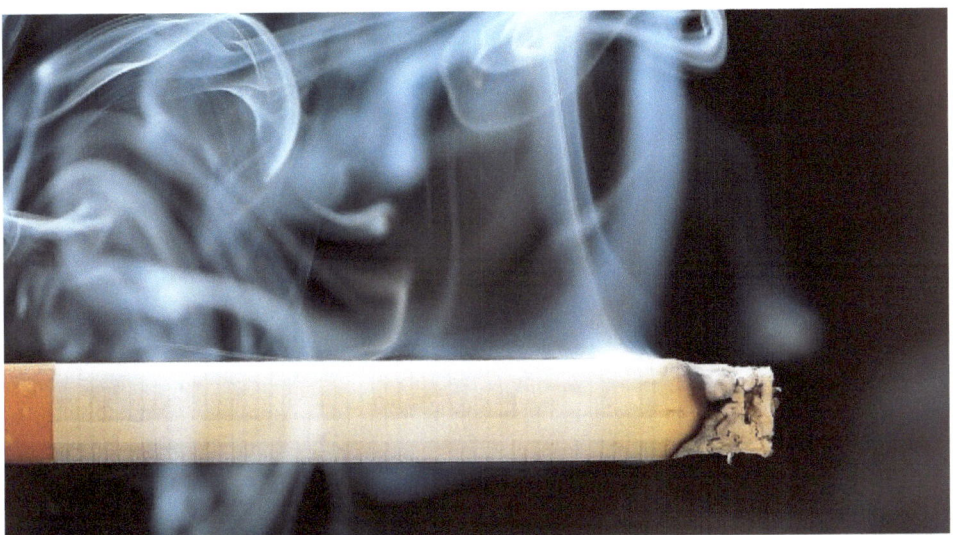

According to a recent study, CBD can be used to help smokers kick the habit. A total of 24 smokers were given an inhaler filled with either CBD or a placebo substance. They were instructed to use the device every time that they got a craving for a cigarette.

Over the course of a week, the CBD group saw a 40% reduction in the frequency of their smoking habit. This had led scientists to believe that CBD could be used as an aid for quitting. If it can be proved that the compound has an impact on cravings for nicotine, the benefits for the medical industry could be huge.

Diabetes

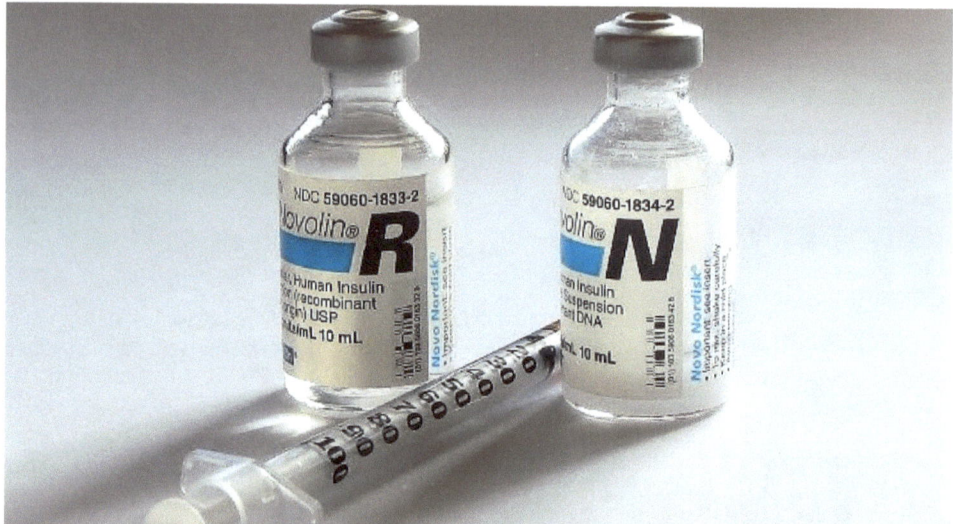

Tests on mice indicate that CBD could be used to prevent or delay the development on Type 1 Diabetes. Though the same effect has not yet been discovered for Type 2 Diabetes (only non-obese mice were prevented from getting the disease), the results are still important.

Treatment with CBD prevented the production of IL-12, from the splenocytes. This is a vital cog in the fight to control and cure diabetes, because restricting the development of this cytokine can alleviate the symptoms of several autoimmune conditions.

Fibromyalgia

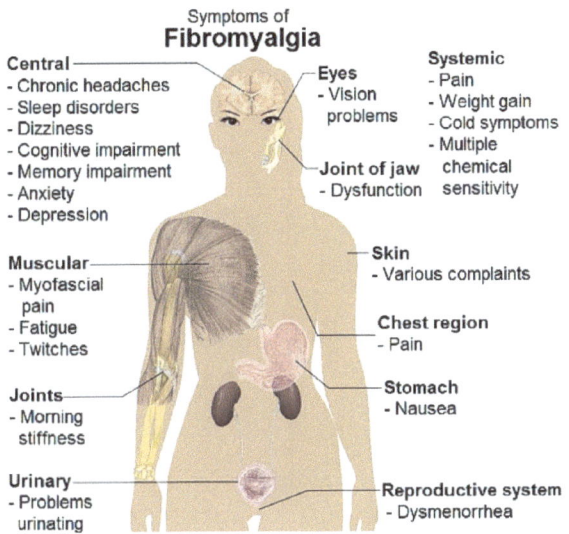

It is common for fibromyalgia to be treated with anti-inflammatory medications, opioid treatments, or corticosteroids. However, a 2011 study, experimented with the use of CBD as a treatment for this condition. The results were very pleasing. Of the 56 study volunteers who were prescribed CBD for their symptoms, all reported some level of reduction.

For the control group, who were not prescribed CBD, there was no reduction in symptoms. Fibromyalgia is a very difficult condition to live with. It causes widespread pain, throughout the body, and makes it hard to stay mobile. If CBD could be used as an effective treatment, in the future, sufferers might be able to improve their quality of life.

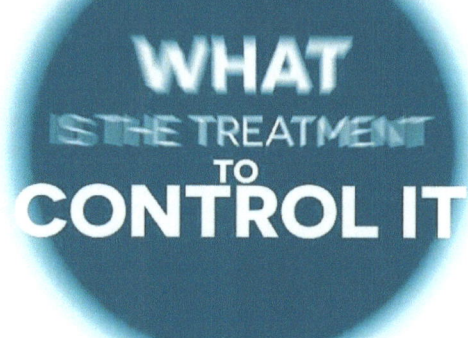

The link between CBD and schizophrenia is an old one. In fact, this mental condition was one of the earliest to be associated with the medical benefits of CBD oil and CBD treatments. The problem, at the moment, is finding a way to amplify and prolong the positive effects of CBD.

Current CBD treatments seem to have quite a short lived effect, so they are not yet a good enough substitute for pharmaceutical options. They do, however, reduce anxiety, restore calm (albeit briefly), and contribute to improved cognitive functioning.

Multiple Sclerosis

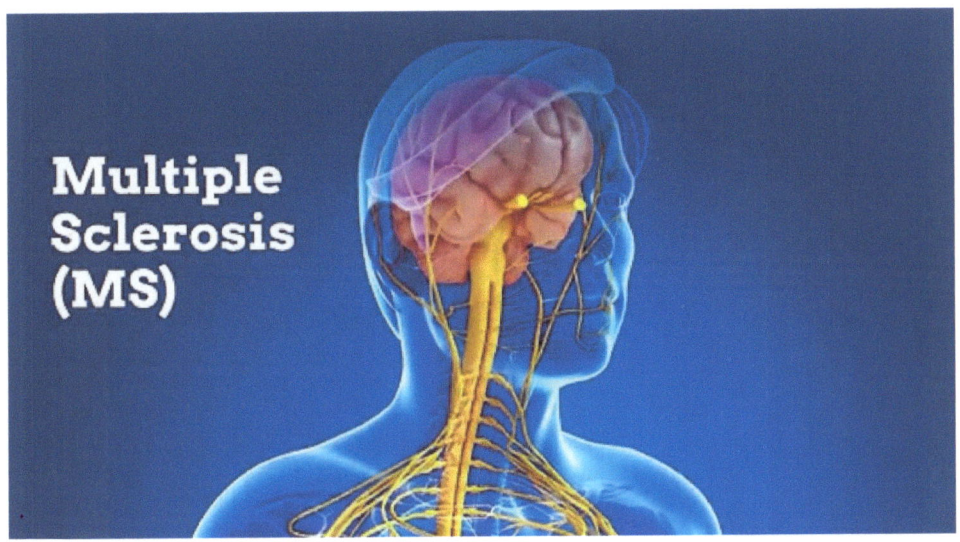

A number of scientists studied animal models and cell cultures to determine that CBD can reverse inflammatory responses and serve as robust protection against the effects of multiple sclerosis. Within ten days, mice treated with CBD exhibited enhanced motor skills and showed a marked progression in their condition.

It is fair to assume then, as these scientists did, that CBD has the potential to reduce a number of aspects of MS. This means that, in the future, it could be used to develop superior treatments and help sufferers deal with the strain that symptoms place on their everyday lives.

Insomnia/Sleep Disorders

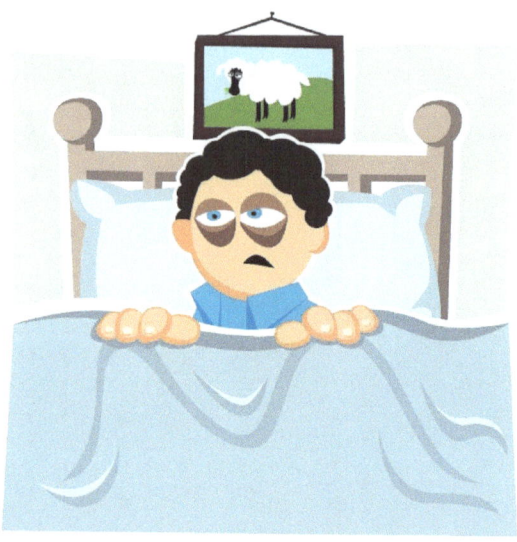

One of the few side effects of CBD is tiredness, but this can be a real advantage for many people. In fact, it is what insomnia sufferers rely on it to do. This is a very important benefit of CBD, because many pharmaceutical treatments for sleep disorders come with the risk of addiction and harmful dependencies.

CBD offers a natural, non-addictive alternative to these options. It is a natural compound, derived from plants, so it has no harmful side effects. Anybody looking for CBD products to alleviate insomnia should search for very heavy strains. On the other hand, for people who don't want this effect, lighter CBD strains can be bought.

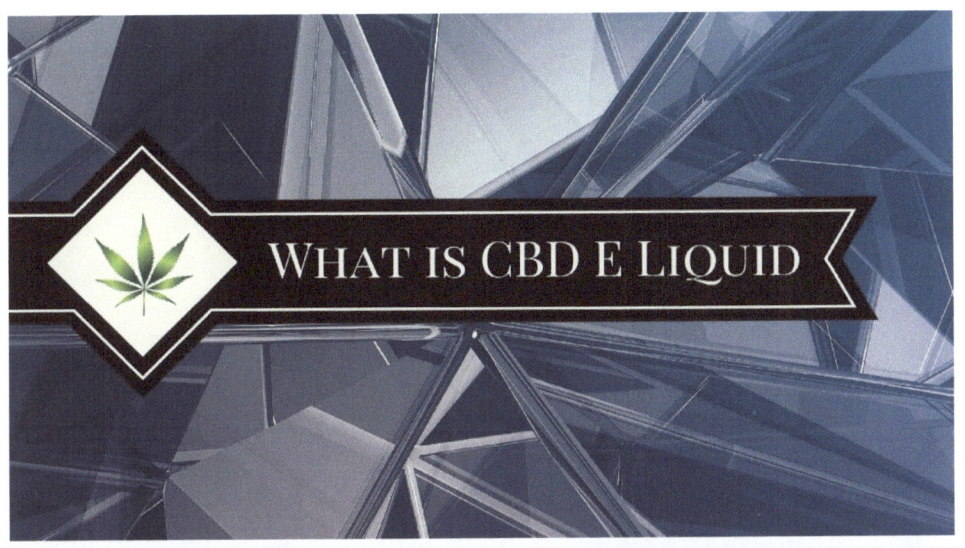

WHAT IS CBD E LIQUID

What is CBD E-Liquid?

CBD e-liquid is CBD oil, in a form that is suitable for use with e-cigarettes and vape sticks and pens. This is a very convenient way to ingest CBD, particularly if a person is used to smoking. While it is not the same as smoking cannabis, it does provide that familiar and comfortable form of intake. For anybody trying to give up regular cigarettes, swapping to a vape pen and CBD e-liquid can make kicking the habit much easier.

These oils and e-liquids work in the same way as standard versions. The vape stick or pen is regularly refilled with the fluid and smoked like cigarette. Most vape pens are now rechargeable or battery powered, so they can be smoked until the power runs down. Then, they can be plugged into a mains supply and powered up again.

CBD e-liquid does not contain any THC. It is legal to buy, use, and distribute in most regions of the world. It is a valuable option for people who like to use CBD, but who are worried about how other people will react to it. Once the liquid is inside the vape stick or pen, there is no way to tell what you are smoking. The e-liquid produces no nasty odors and it can be ingested in public without causing any kind of fuss or inconvenience to others.

In fact, smoking CBD e-liquid is a lot safer than smoking regular cigarettes, for both the user and the people around them. There are no harmful toxins, chemicals, or poisonous compounds in these fluids. They are sold in small bottles, at an affordable price, both in stores and online. Before buying CBD e-liquids from an online vendor, check for customer reviews and testimonials.

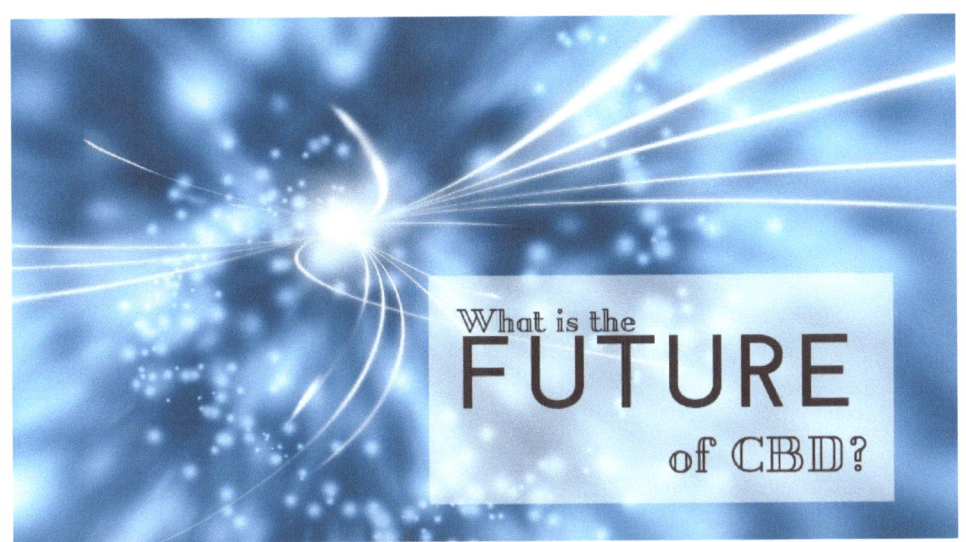

What is the Future of CBD?

Fortunately, the future looks very bright for CBD and its potential uses within the medical industry. As scientists and medical researchers grow more comfortable with its association with the cannabis plant, they will inevitably become more willing to explore its properties. This is good news not just for those with multiple sclerosis, schizophrenia, and sleep disorders, but also for anybody who prefers to rely on natural medicines.

The benefits of CBD are becoming harder to ignore. It is quite clear what it can do. All that remains now is to embrace its use and work out what kind of applications it has for both mild and more comprehensive treatments. People interested in trying CBD for the first time should not shy away from the opportunity. It is safe, side effect free, and could just change your life.

Source - http://cannabiscbdoil.org/

www.ingramcontent.com/pod-product-compliance
Lightning Source LLC
Chambersburg PA
CBHW050909290526
45792CB00002B/756